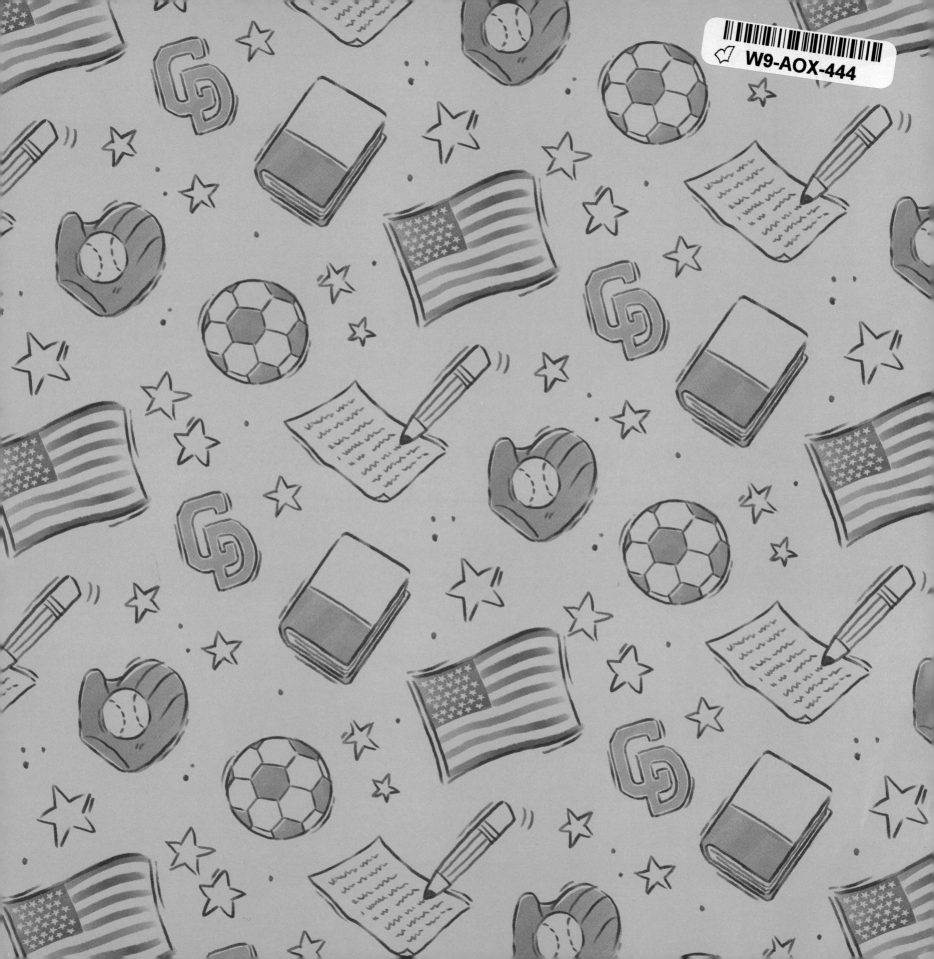

This book is dedicated to all the children that are going through something difficult. Your imperfections are your gifts. I also dedicate this book to all the people who have supported me. I also dedicate my book to my dog, Caitin. She was there for me whenever I felt down. I couldn't have accepted my stutter without you.—B.H.

For Andy, the wind beneath my wings.—B.C.T.

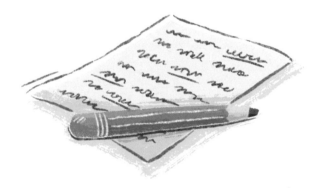

Special thanks to David Ritz

Brayden Speaks Up
Text copyright © 2021 by Brayden Harrington
Illustrations copyright © 2021 by Betty C. Tang
All rights reserved. Printed in the United States of America.
No part of this book may be used or reproduced in any manner whatsoever without written permission except in the case of brief quotations embodied in critical articles and reviews. For information address HarperCollins Children's Books, a division of HarperCollins Publishers, 195 Broadway, New York, NY 10007.
www.harpercollinschildrens.com

ISBN 978-0-06-309829-9

The artist used Procreate and Clip Studio Paint to create the digital illustrations for this book.
Typography by Caitlin Stamper
21 22 23 24 25 PC 10 9 8 7 6 5 4 3 2 1
❖
First Edition

BRAYDEN HARRINGTON
BRAYDEN SPEAKS UP

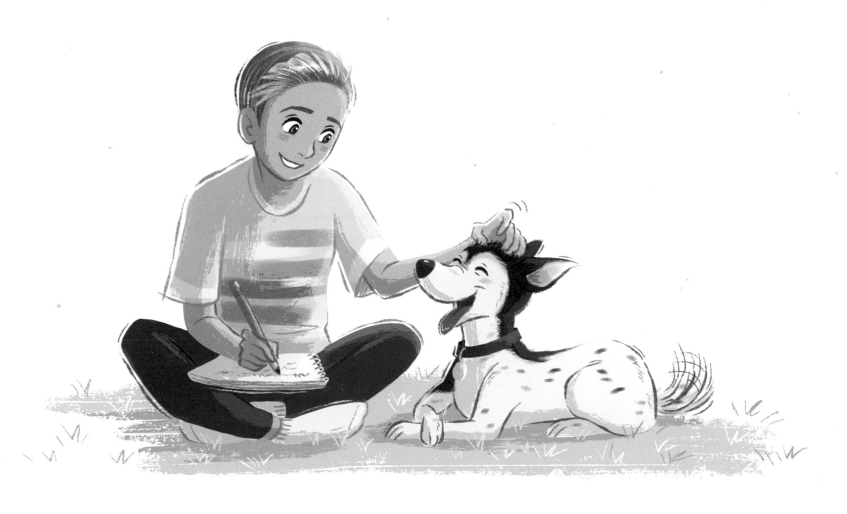

Illustrated by Betty C. Tang

HARPER
An Imprint of HarperCollinsPublishers

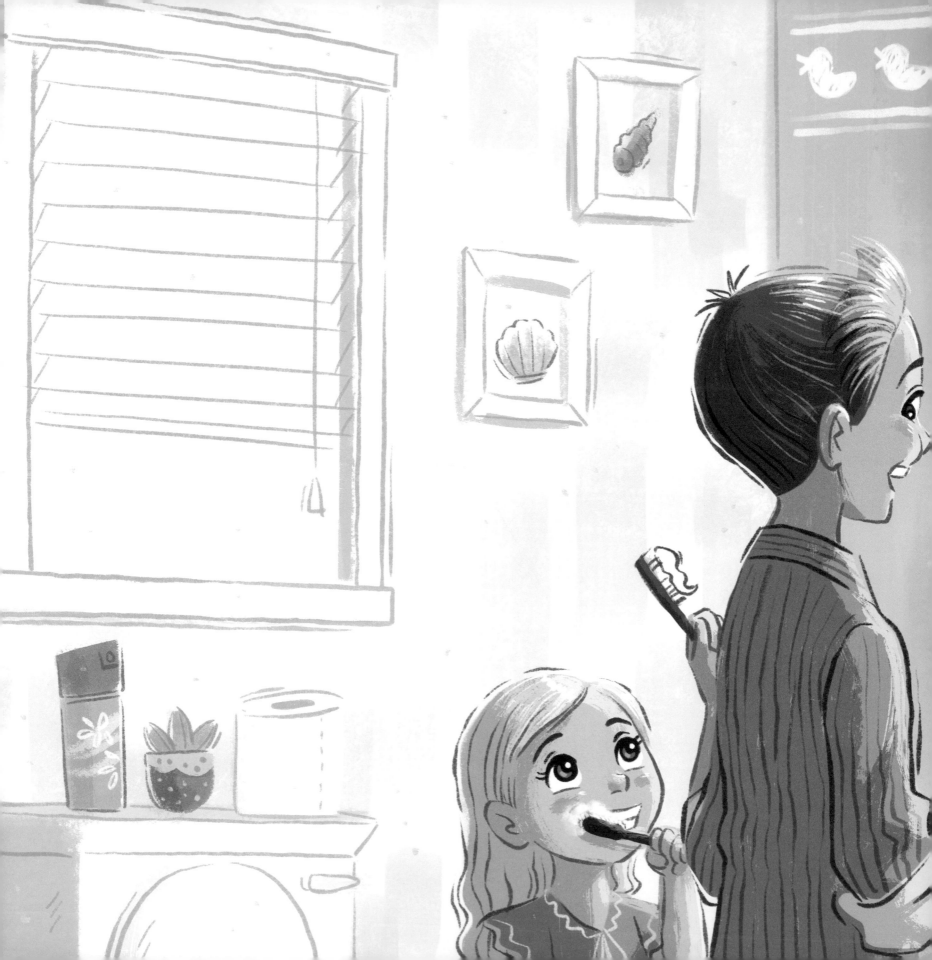

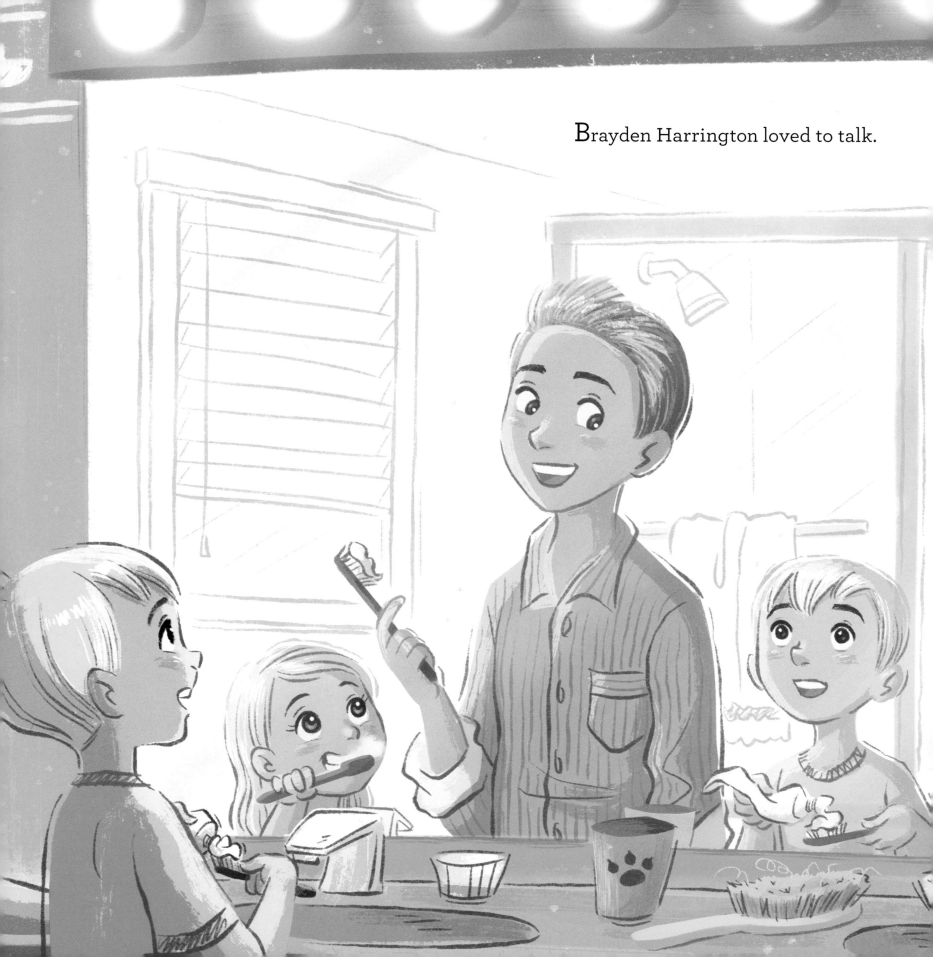

Brayden Harrington loved to talk.

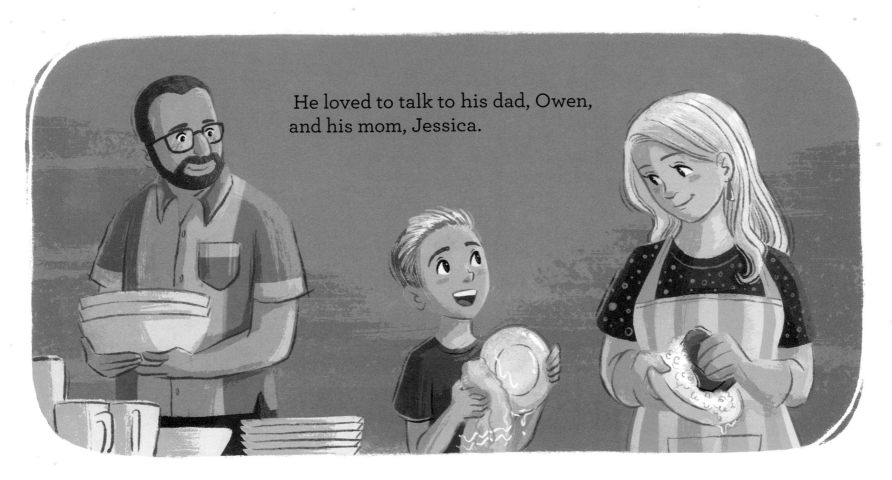

He loved to talk to his dad, Owen, and his mom, Jessica.

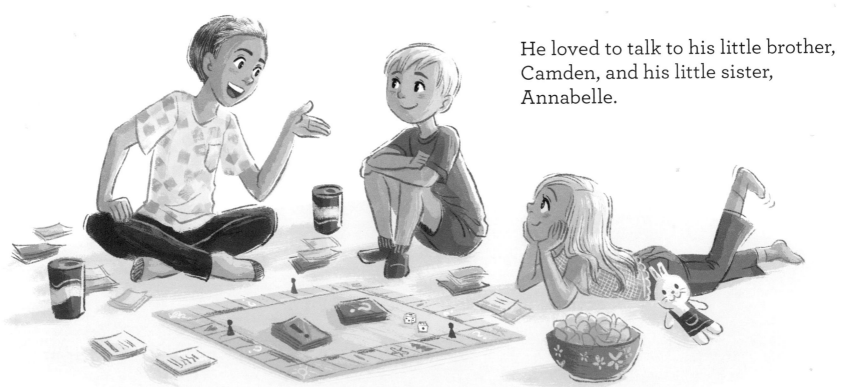

He loved to talk to his little brother, Camden, and his little sister, Annabelle.

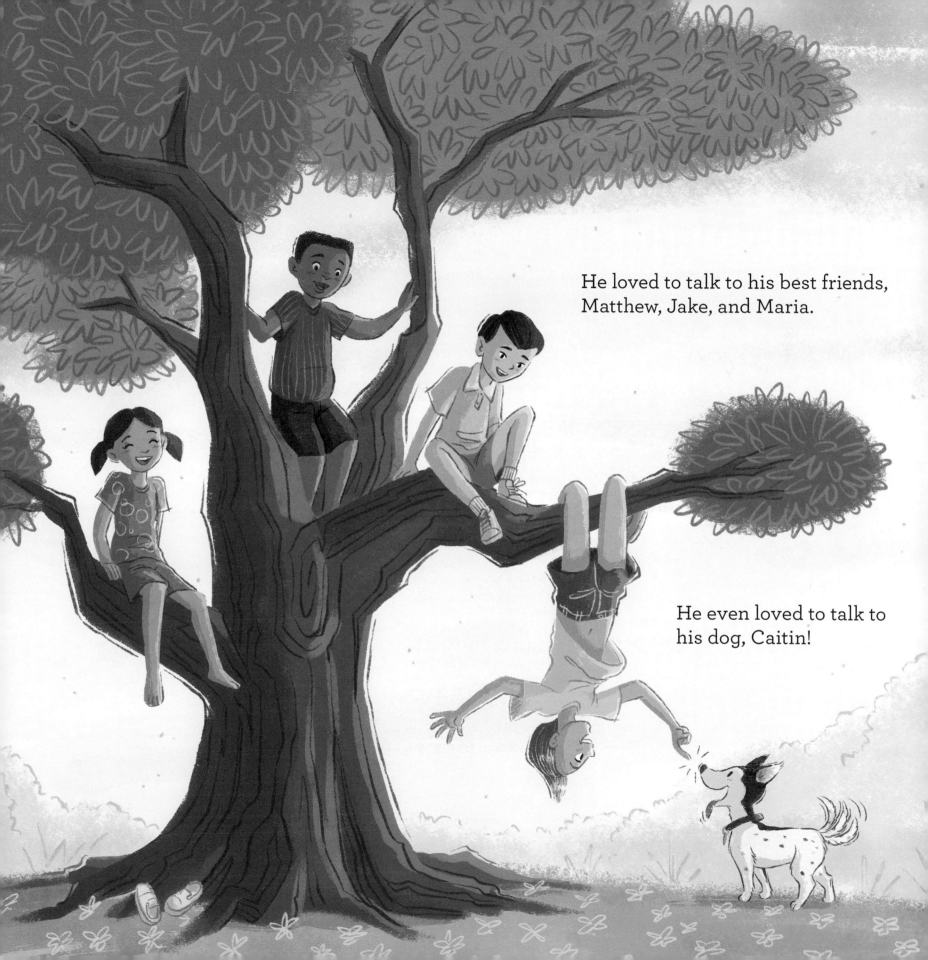

He loved to talk to his best friends, Matthew, Jake, and Maria.

He even loved to talk to his dog, Caitin!

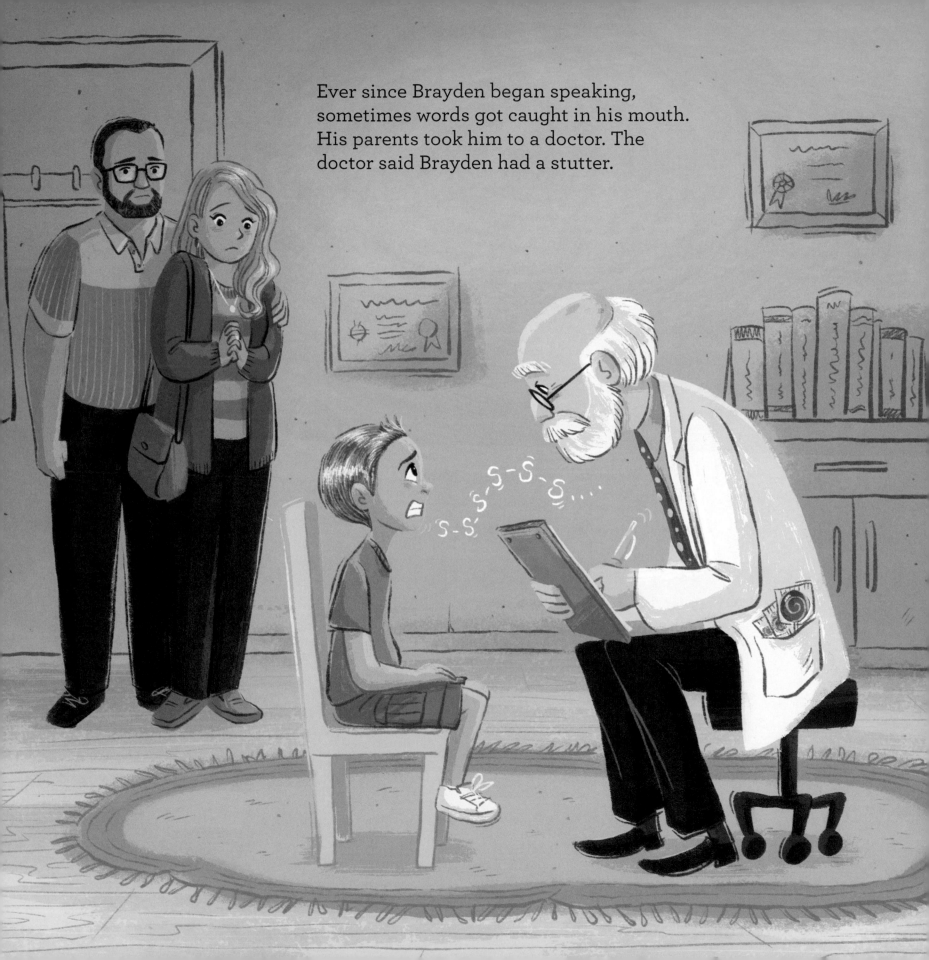

Ever since Brayden began speaking, sometimes words got caught in his mouth. His parents took him to a doctor. The doctor said Brayden had a stutter.

"You have bumpy speech,"
Brayden's mom said.
"And that's okay!"

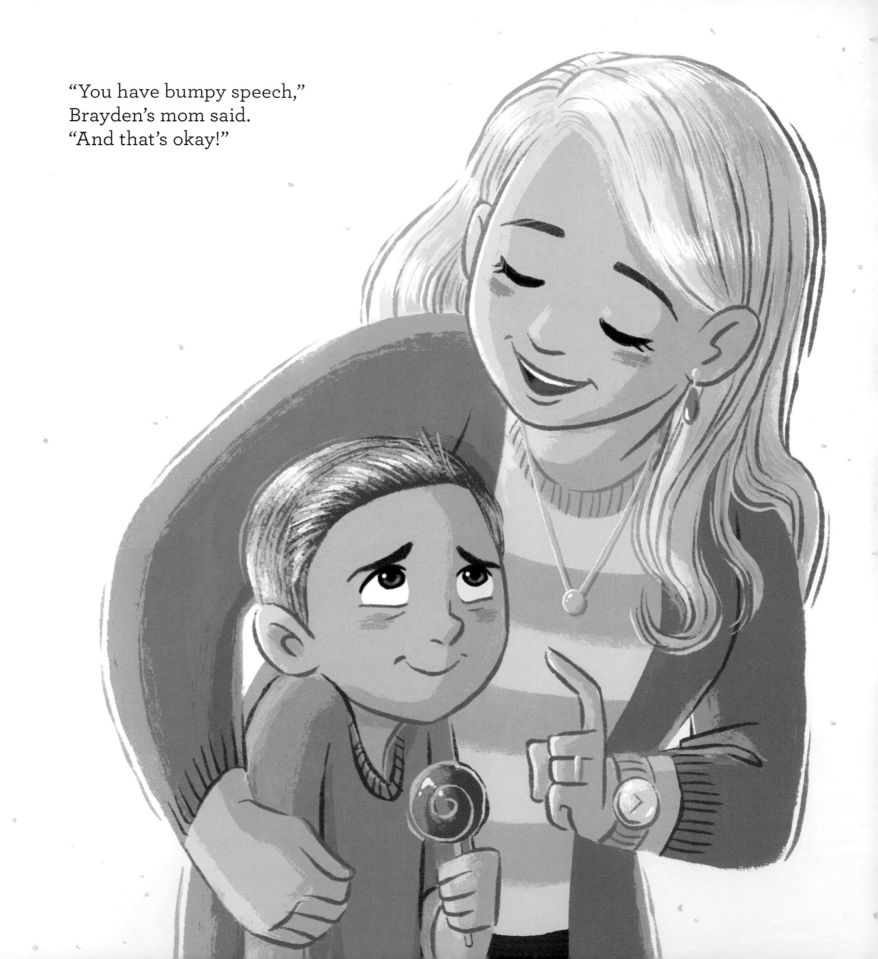

Brayden didn't mind his bumpy speech. Except when his words got stuck at embarrassing moments. One time a teacher asked Brayden to name the capital of their state, New Hampshire. He knew the answer right away.

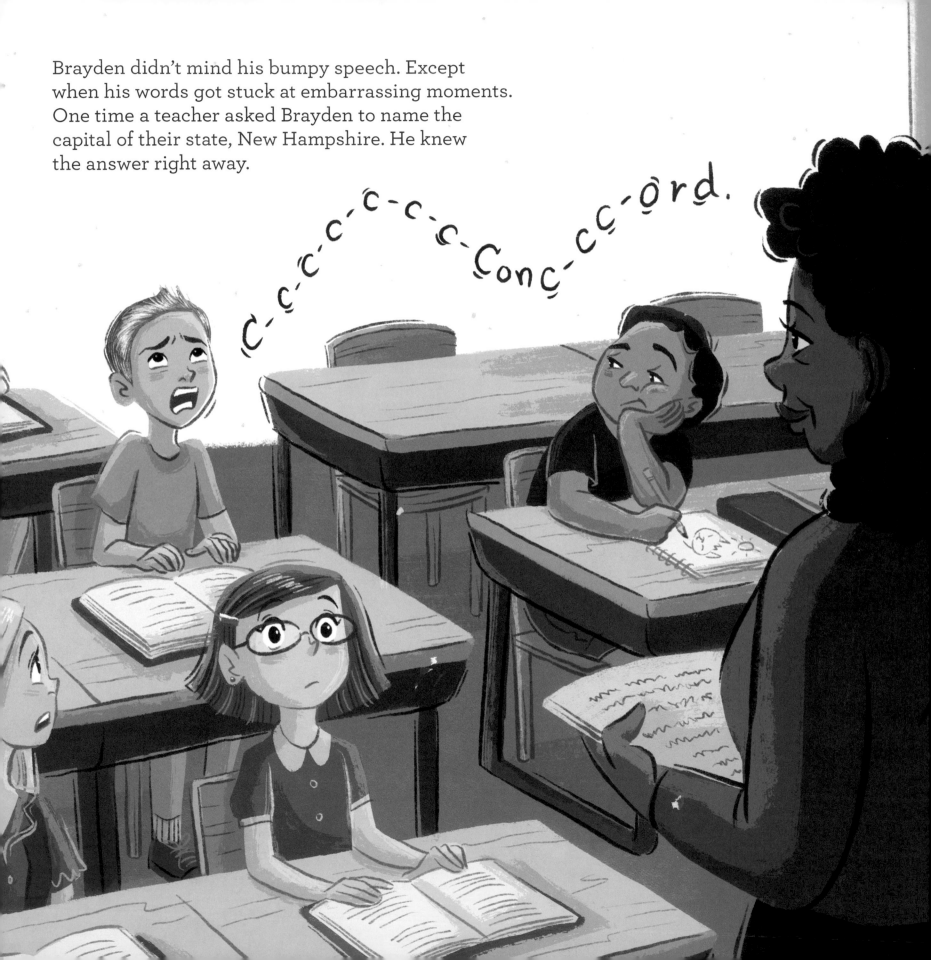

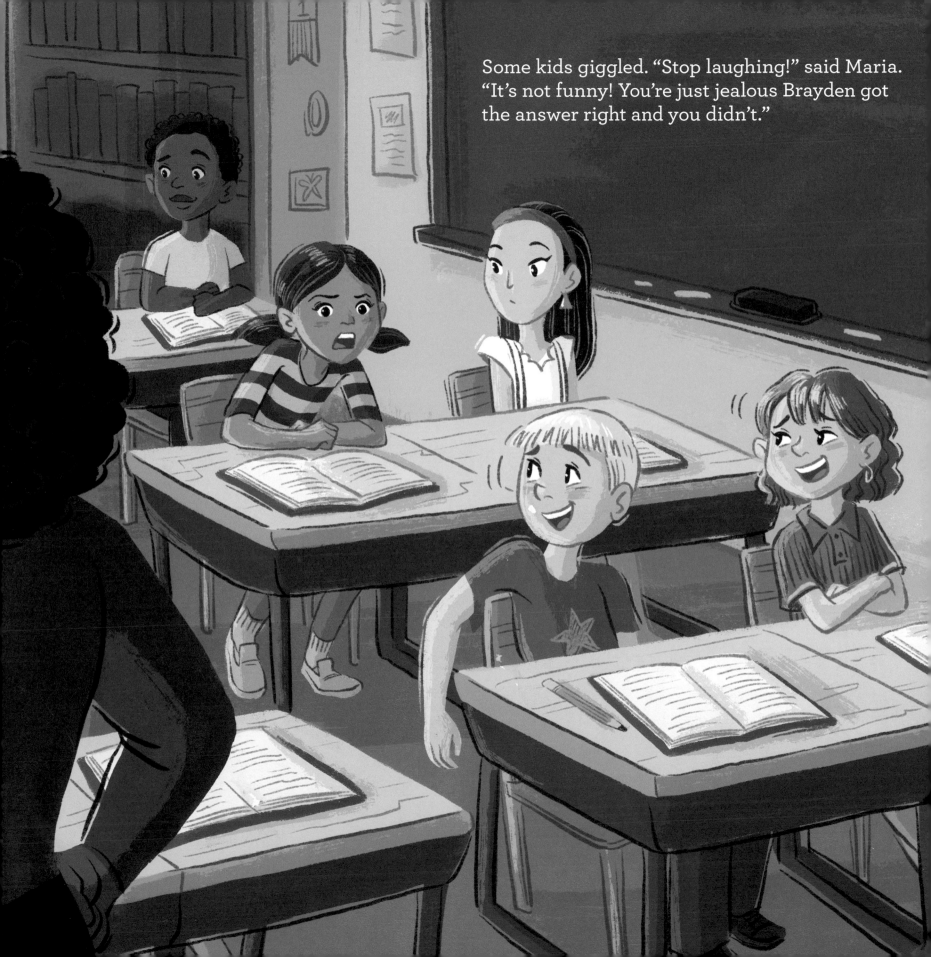

Some kids giggled. "Stop laughing!" said Maria. "It's not funny! You're just jealous Brayden got the answer right and you didn't."

And when Brayden felt pressure, his speech got bumpier. Like the time his teacher announced that everyone in his grade had to memorize the Gettysburg Address. Brayden was a little worried.

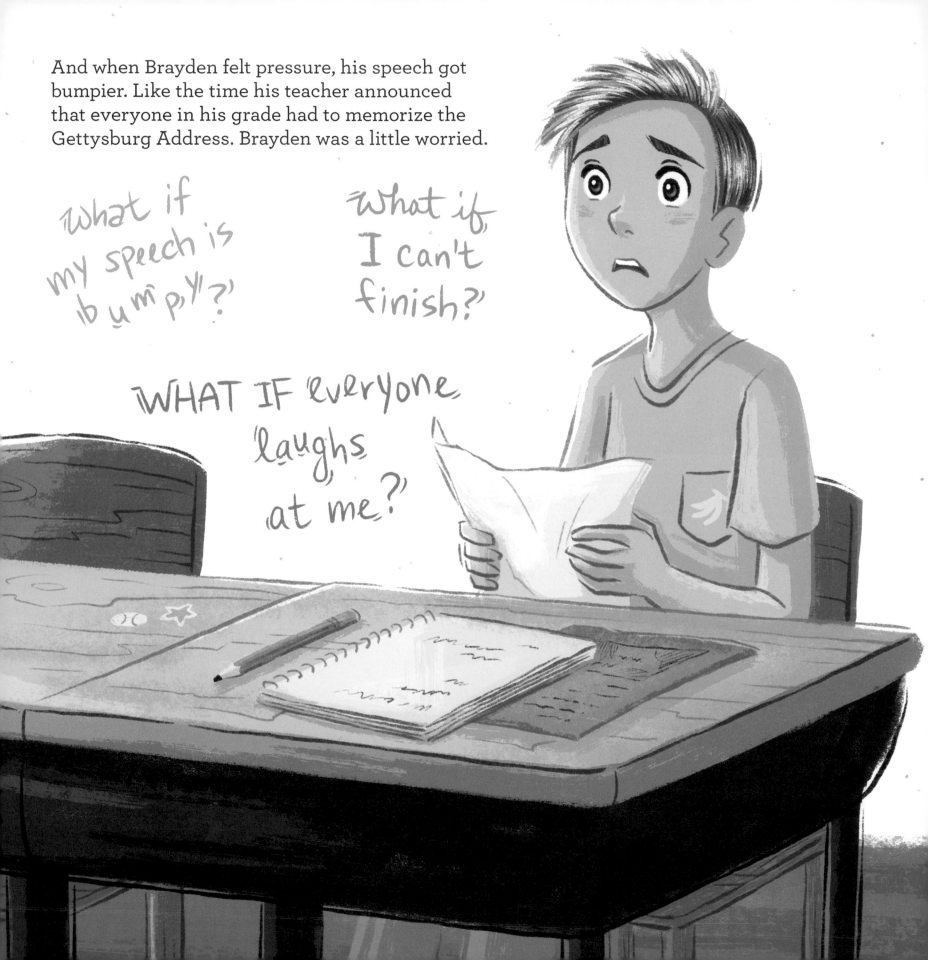

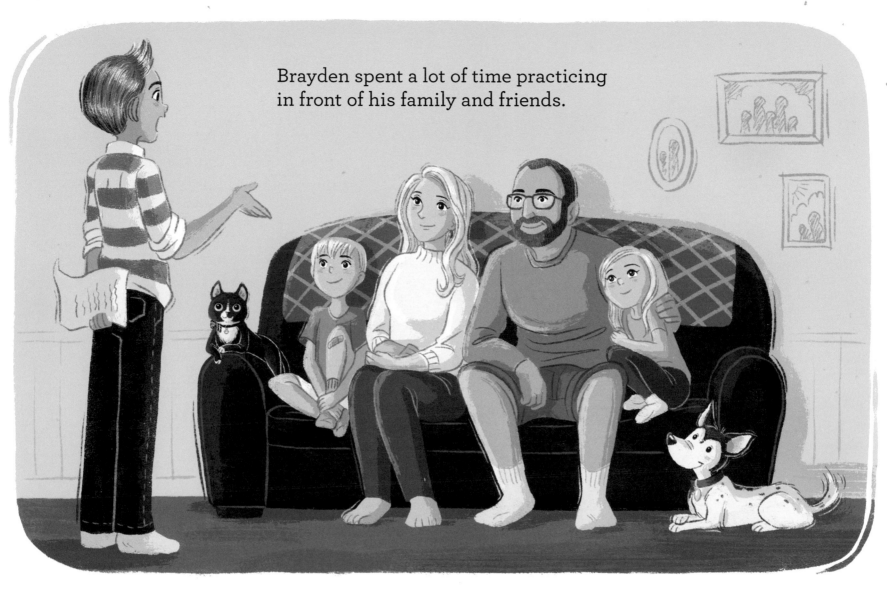

Brayden spent a lot of time practicing in front of his family and friends.

"You'll do great, Brayden!" they said.

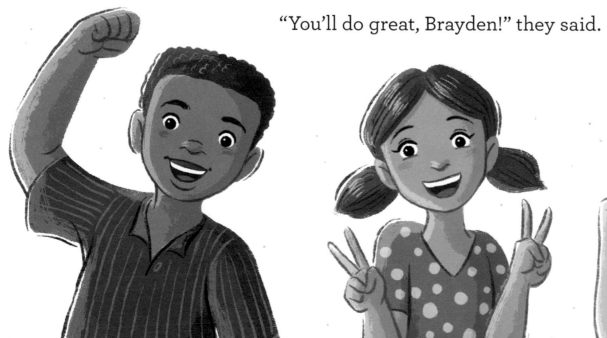
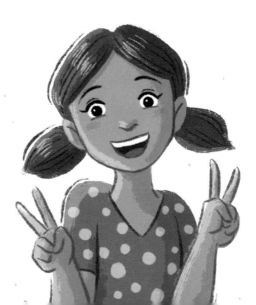
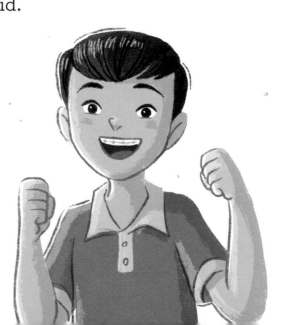

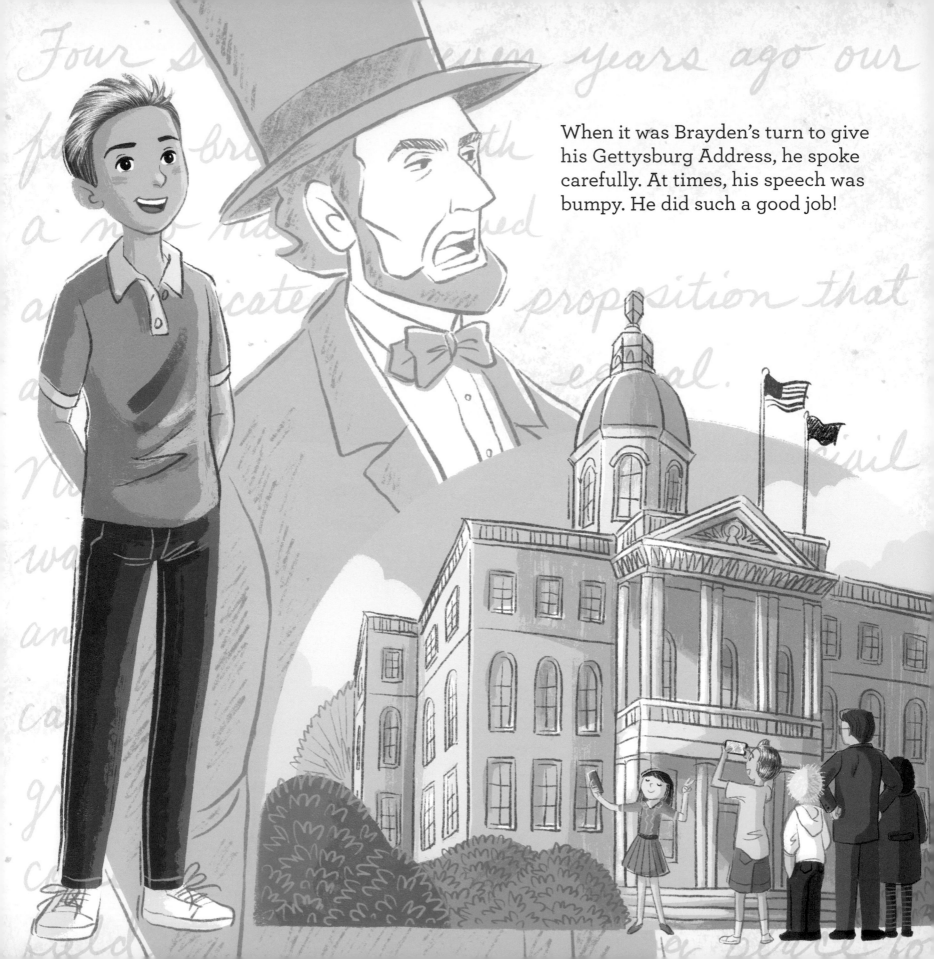

When it was Brayden's turn to give his Gettysburg Address, he spoke carefully. At times, his speech was bumpy. He did such a good job!

Along with several other classmates, Brayden was chosen to tour the State House and eat dinner at a fancy restaurant.

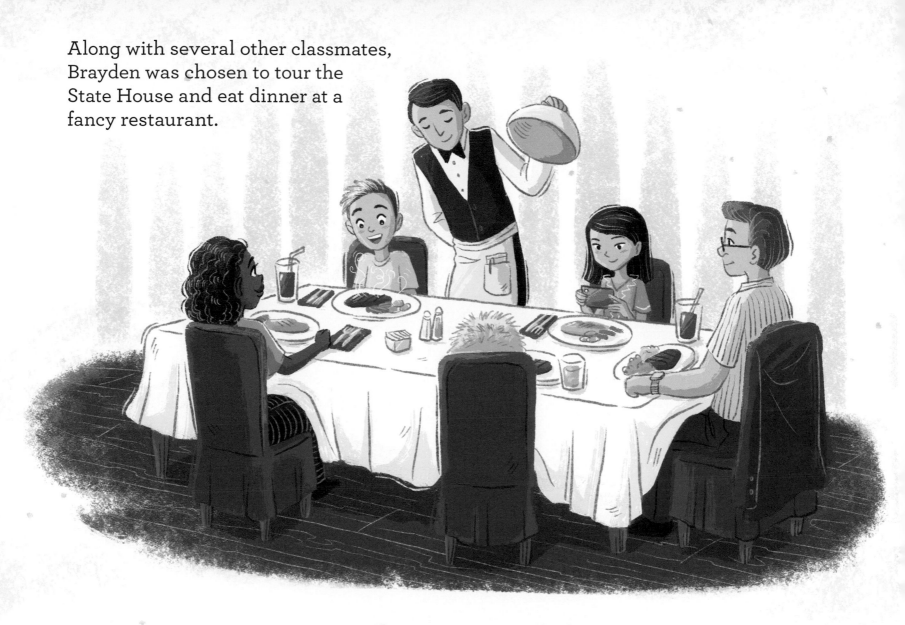

They even got to ride there in a big limo!

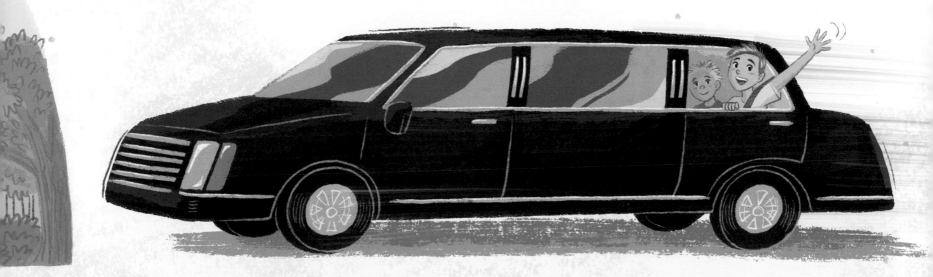

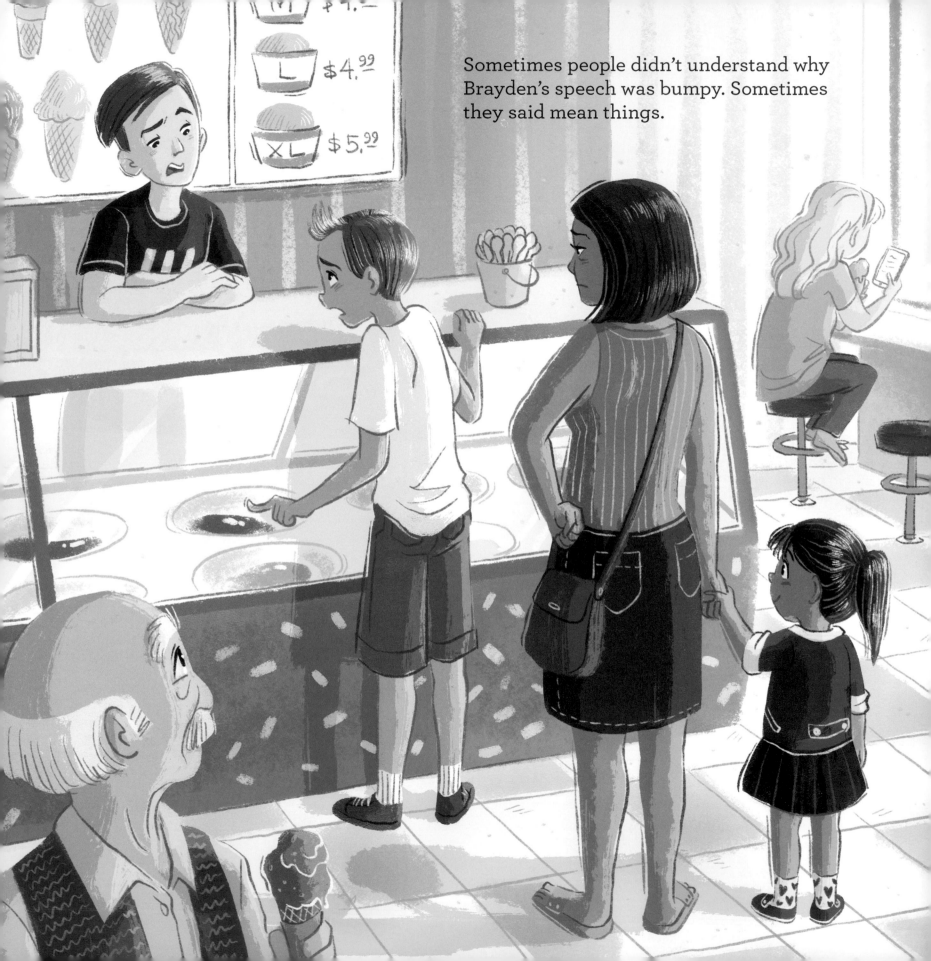

Sometimes people didn't understand why Brayden's speech was bumpy. Sometimes they said mean things.

But Brayden never let anyone keep him down. And his best friends were always there for him.

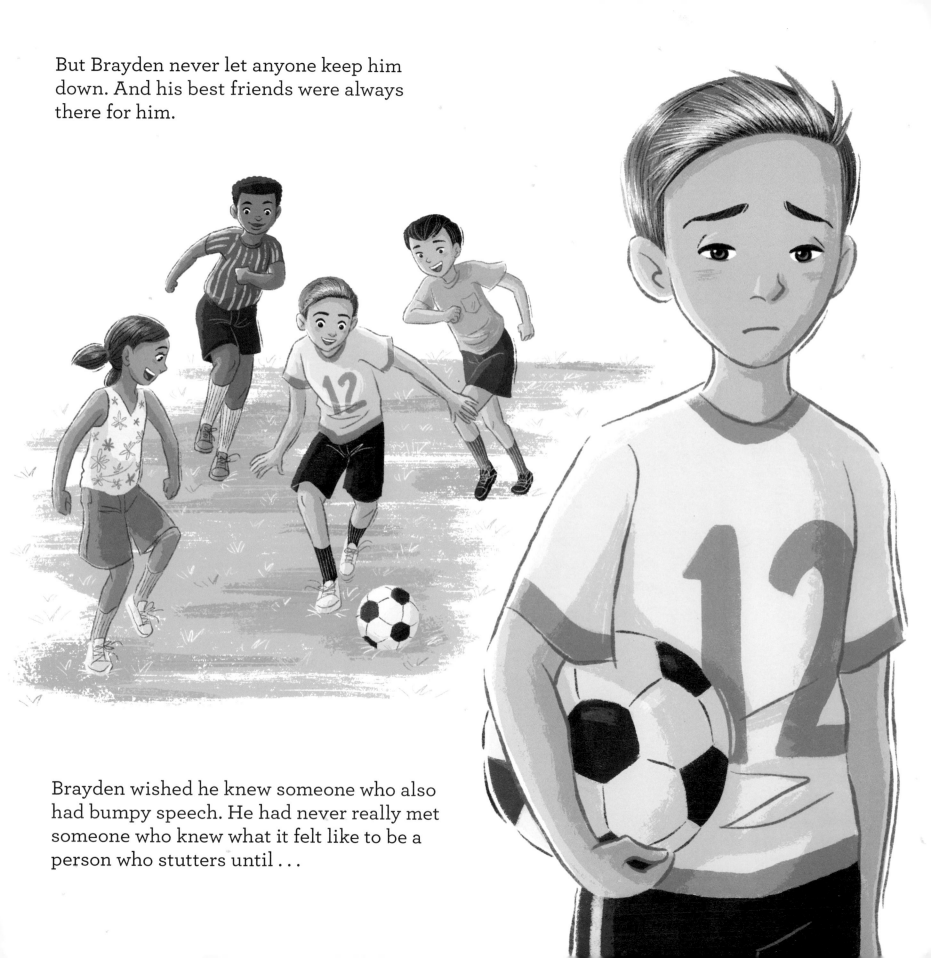

Brayden wished he knew someone who also had bumpy speech. He had never really met someone who knew what it felt like to be a person who stutters until . . .

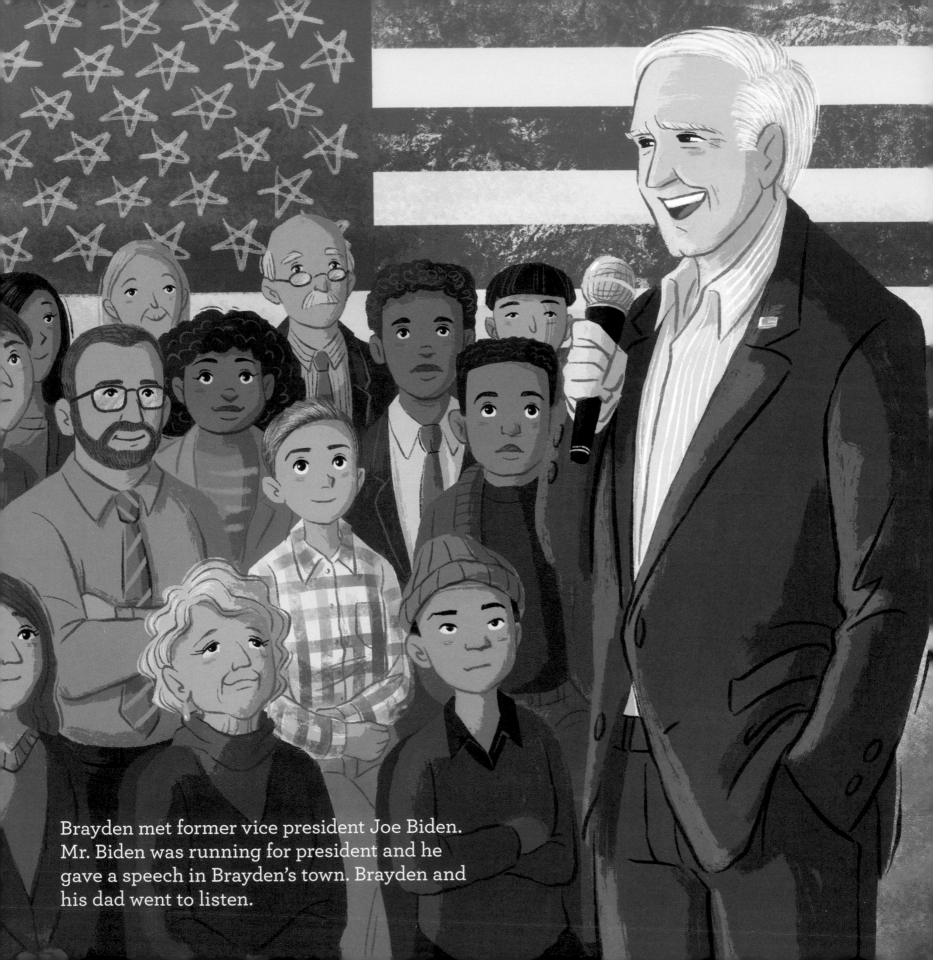

Brayden met former vice president Joe Biden.
Mr. Biden was running for president and he
gave a speech in Brayden's town. Brayden and
his dad went to listen.

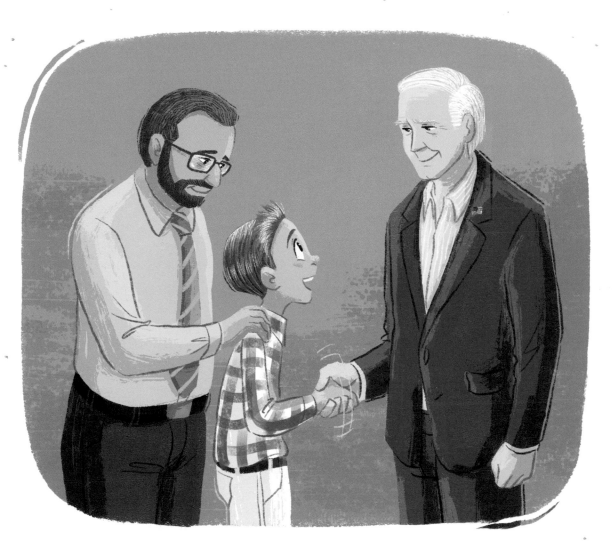

After, they got to meet Mr. Biden. Brayden was so excited he couldn't speak. Brayden's dad explained that sometimes Brayden's words got stuck because he had bumpy speech. "That's okay," said Mr. Biden. "When I was your age, I had bumpy speech, too."

Brayden couldn't believe it. Someone who stuttered like him could be the next president of the United States!

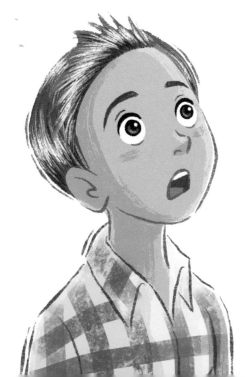

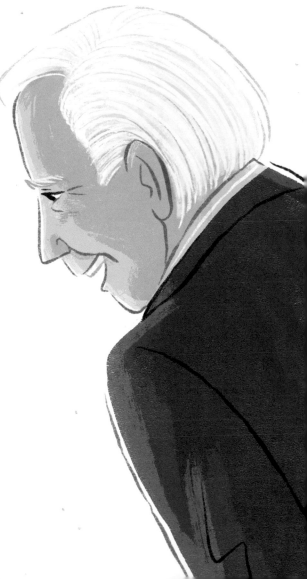

Mr. Biden talked with Brayden for a long time.
"My bumpy speech didn't stop me.
Nothing should stop you."

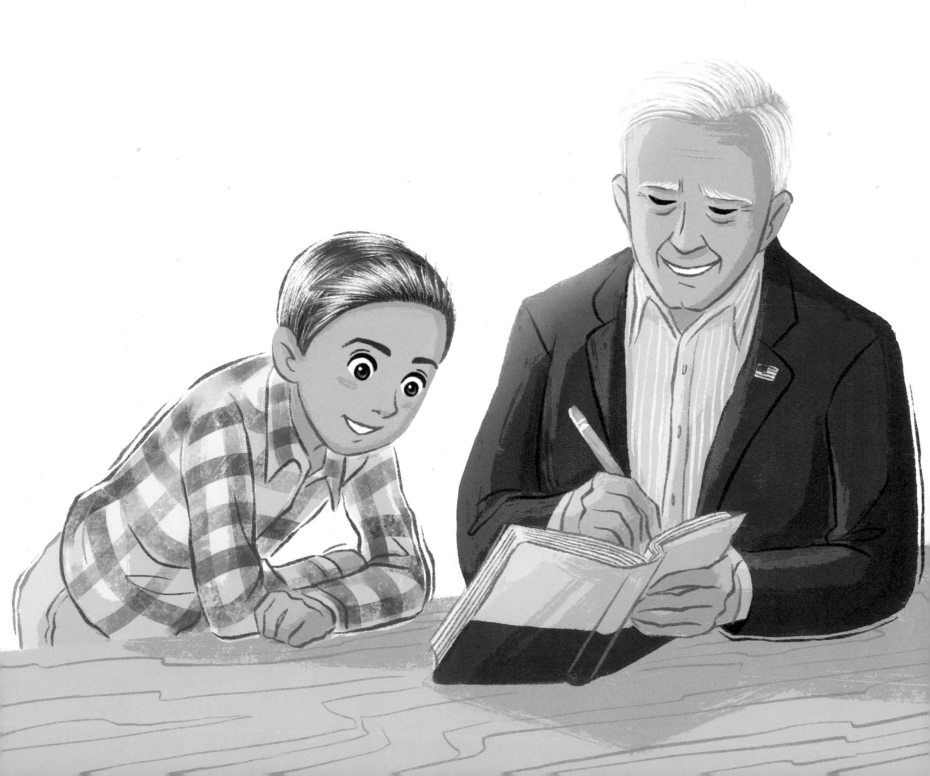

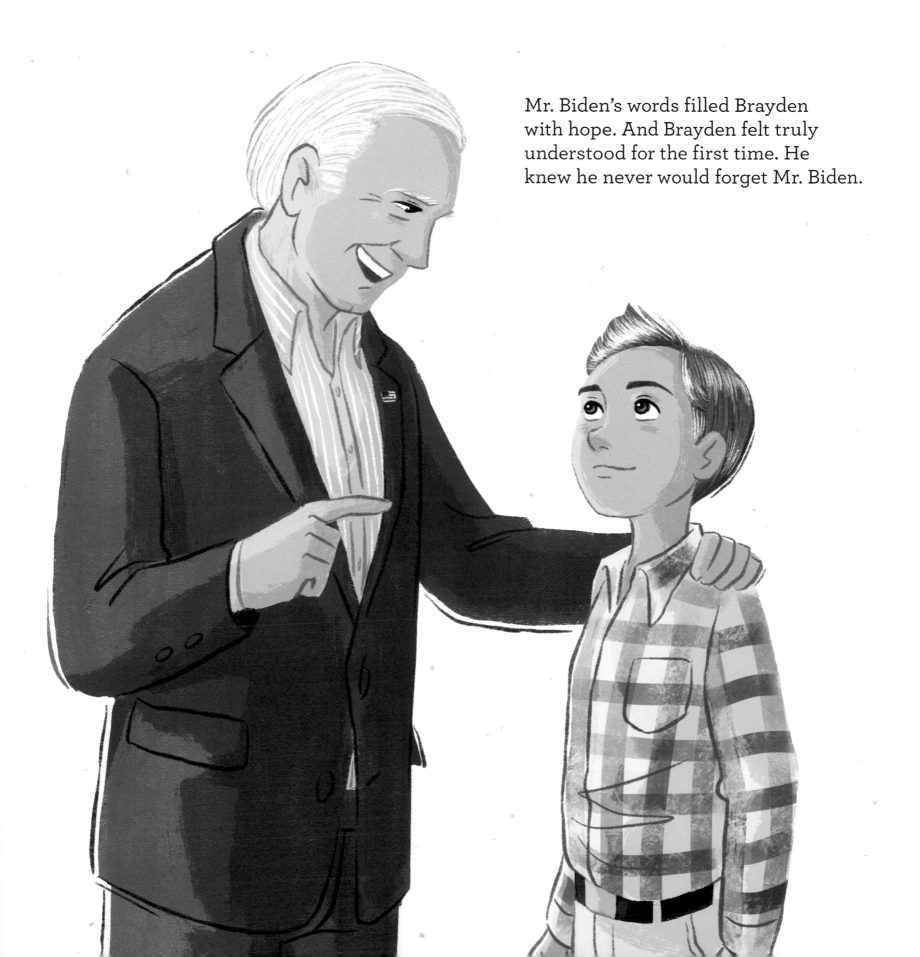

Mr. Biden's words filled Brayden with hope. And Brayden felt truly understood for the first time. He knew he never would forget Mr. Biden.

A few weeks later, Mr. Biden's team asked Brayden to talk on TV at the Democratic National Convention! Millions of people would be watching this big speech.

Brayden was nervous. But his family and friends encouraged him. He agreed to do it.

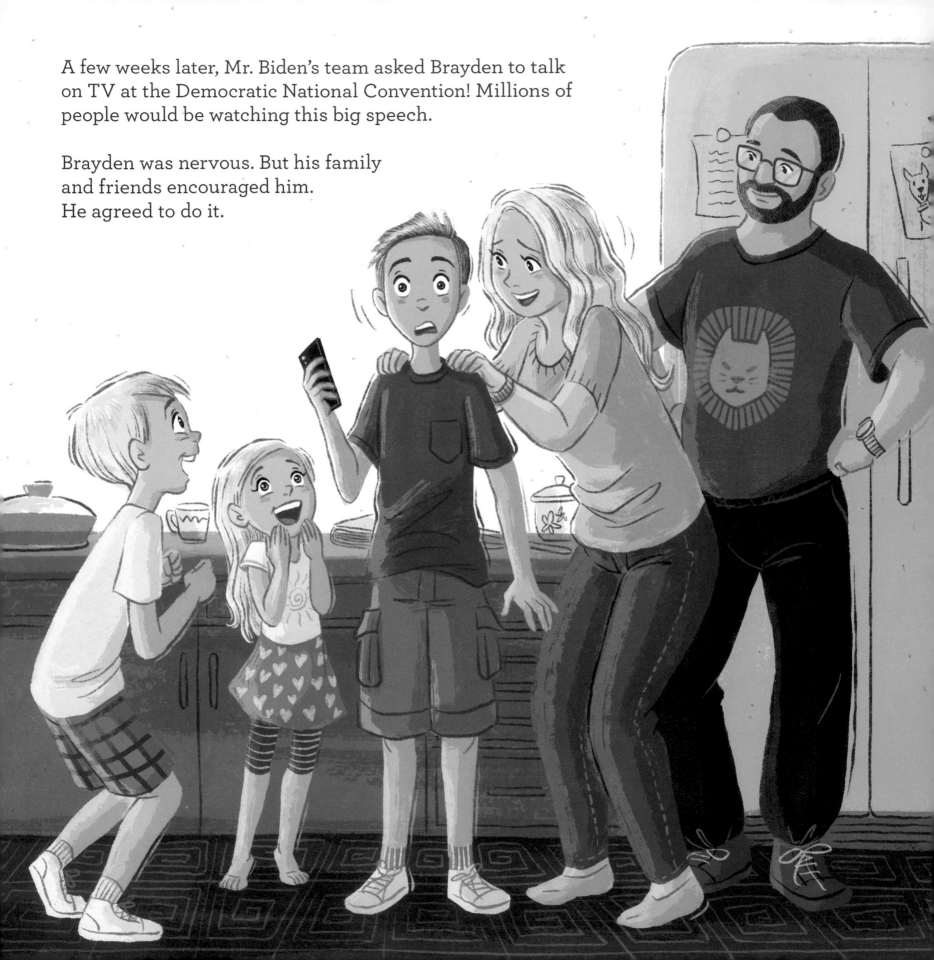

Brayden started working on what he was going to say.
"We all want the world to feel better, Brayden," Annabelle said.
"You can help do that."
What a great line for his speech!

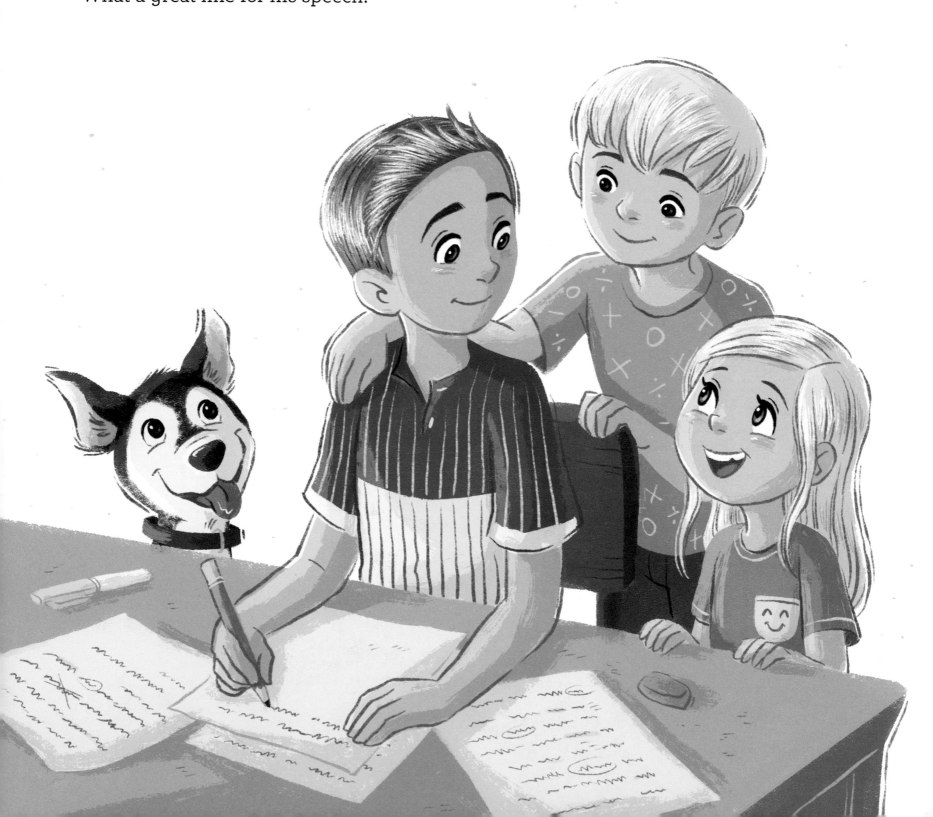

When the big day arrived, Brayden was ready. But he was still nervous. His what-ifs grew louder and scarier than they ever had before.

What if my speech is so bumpy I can't finish?

What if everyone laughs at me?

WHAT IF I let everyone down?

What if?

WHAT IF?

What if?

what if?

what if?

what if?

He began to cry.

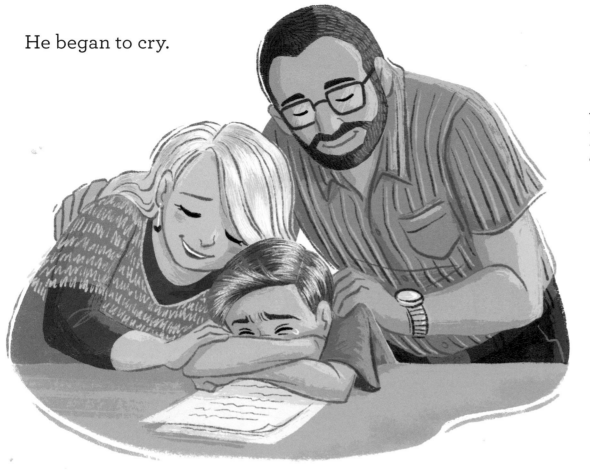

"You don't have to do this if you don't want to, Brayden," his parents said. "It's up to you."

This would be the scariest thing Brayden had *ever* done in his life. There would be a lot of pressure and his speech would be bumpy. But then Brayden thought about other kids like him—kids with bumpy speech. By going on TV, maybe he could give them hope. The way Joe Biden had done for him.

Brayden knew what he had to do. "I'll give the speech!" he said, wiping away his tears.

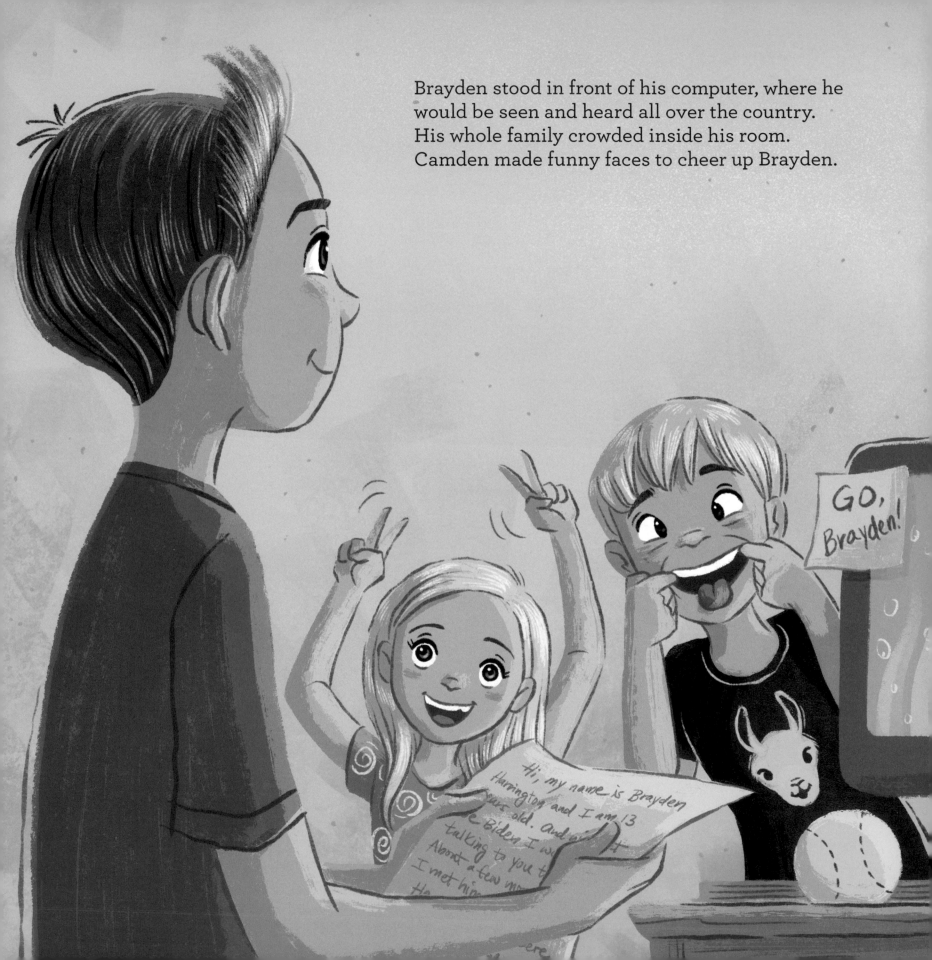

Brayden stood in front of his computer, where he would be seen and heard all over the country. His whole family crowded inside his room. Camden made funny faces to cheer up Brayden.

With his family by his side, Brayden could do this!

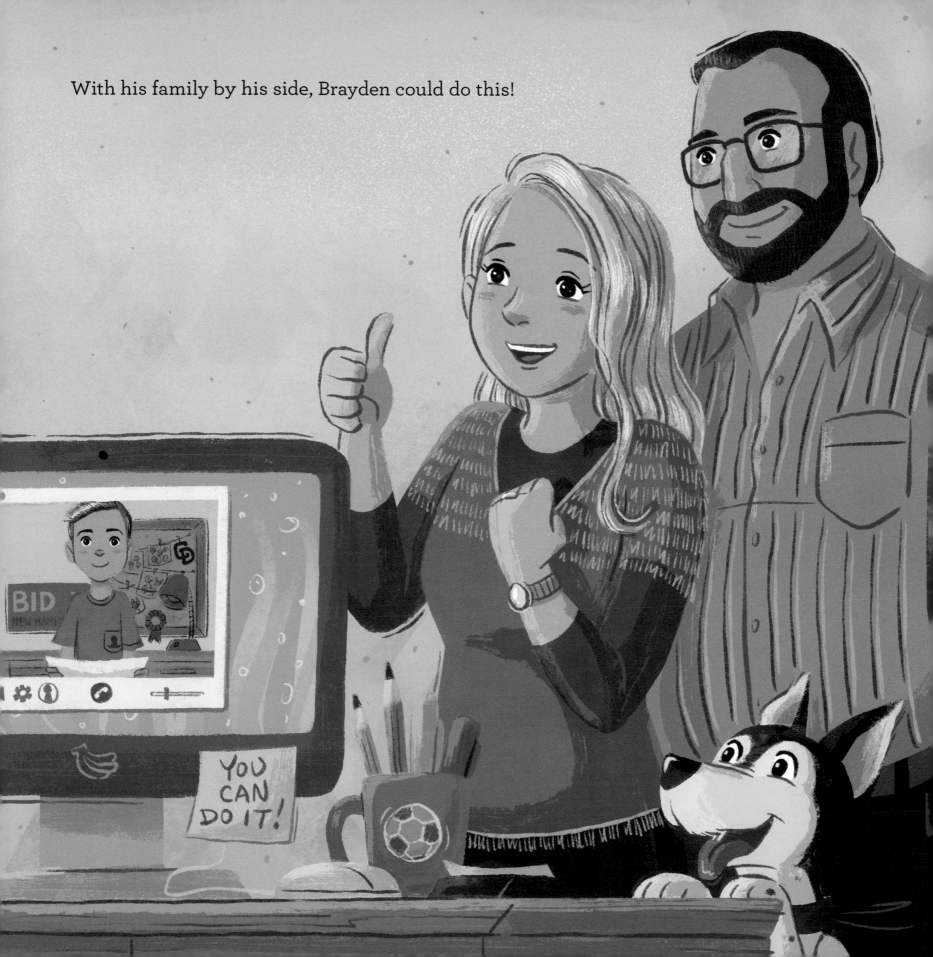

Finally, it was time. Taking a deep breath, Brayden started to talk. His words were not bumpy at first.

"Hi, my name is Brayden Harrington and I'm thirteen years old. And without Joe Biden I wouldn't be talking to you today. About a few months ago, I met him in New Hampshire. He told me that we were members of the same club. We s-s-s-s- . . . S-s-s-s- . . .

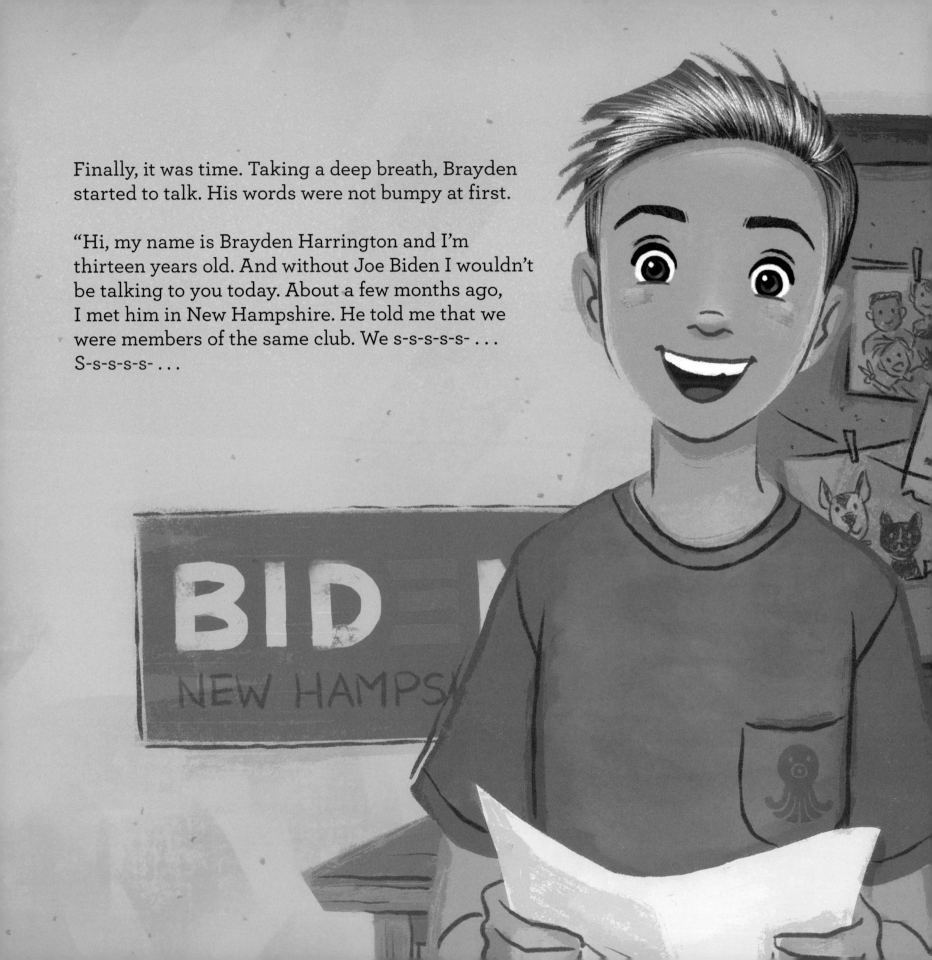

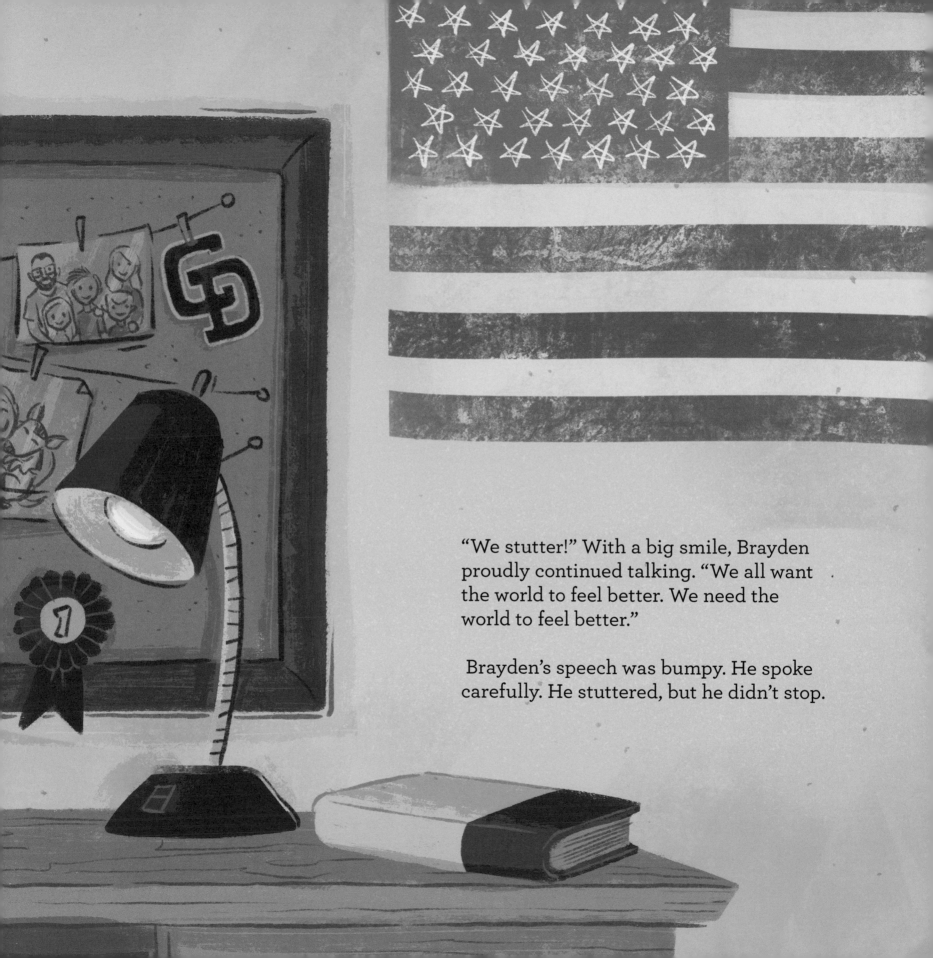

"We stutter!" With a big smile, Brayden proudly continued talking. "We all want the world to feel better. We need the world to feel better."

Brayden's speech was bumpy. He spoke carefully. He stuttered, but he didn't stop.

People all over the world loved Brayden's big speech.

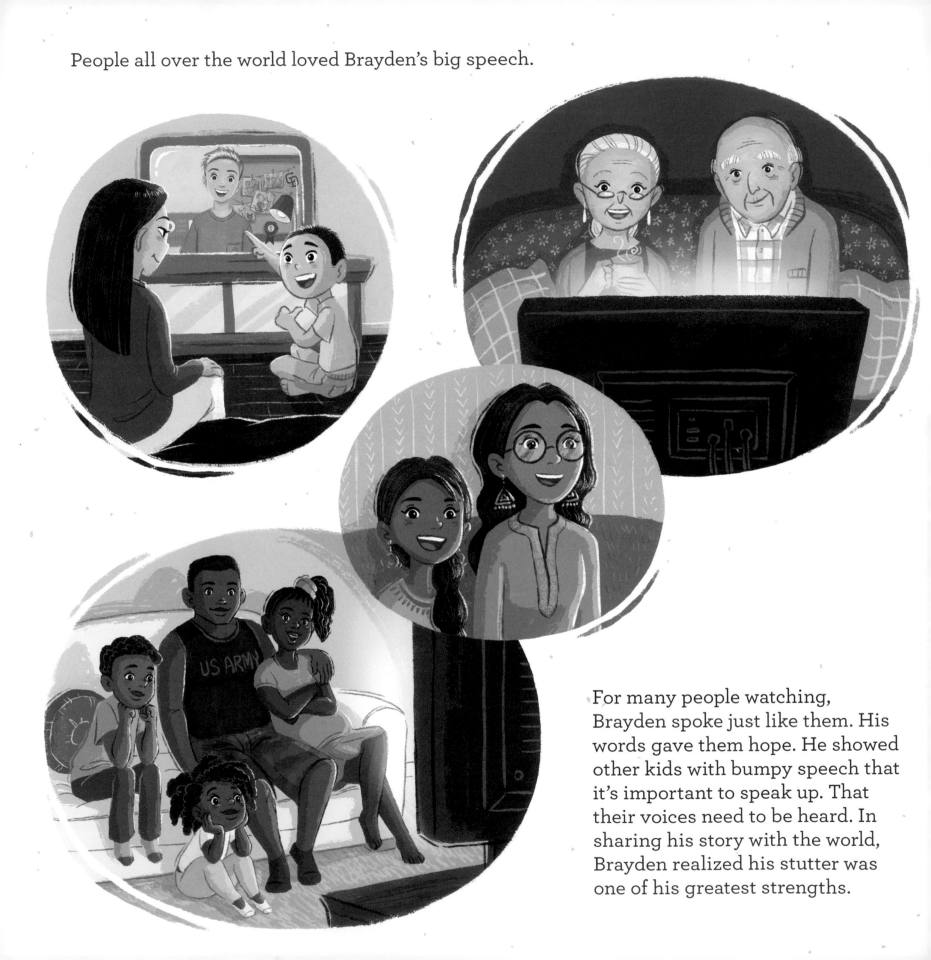

For many people watching, Brayden spoke just like them. His words gave them hope. He showed other kids with bumpy speech that it's important to speak up. That their voices need to be heard. In sharing his story with the world, Brayden realized his stutter was one of his greatest strengths.

Brayden's family and friends were so proud of him.
Messages of praise flooded in, and soon everyone
wanted to talk to Brayden!
And then . . .

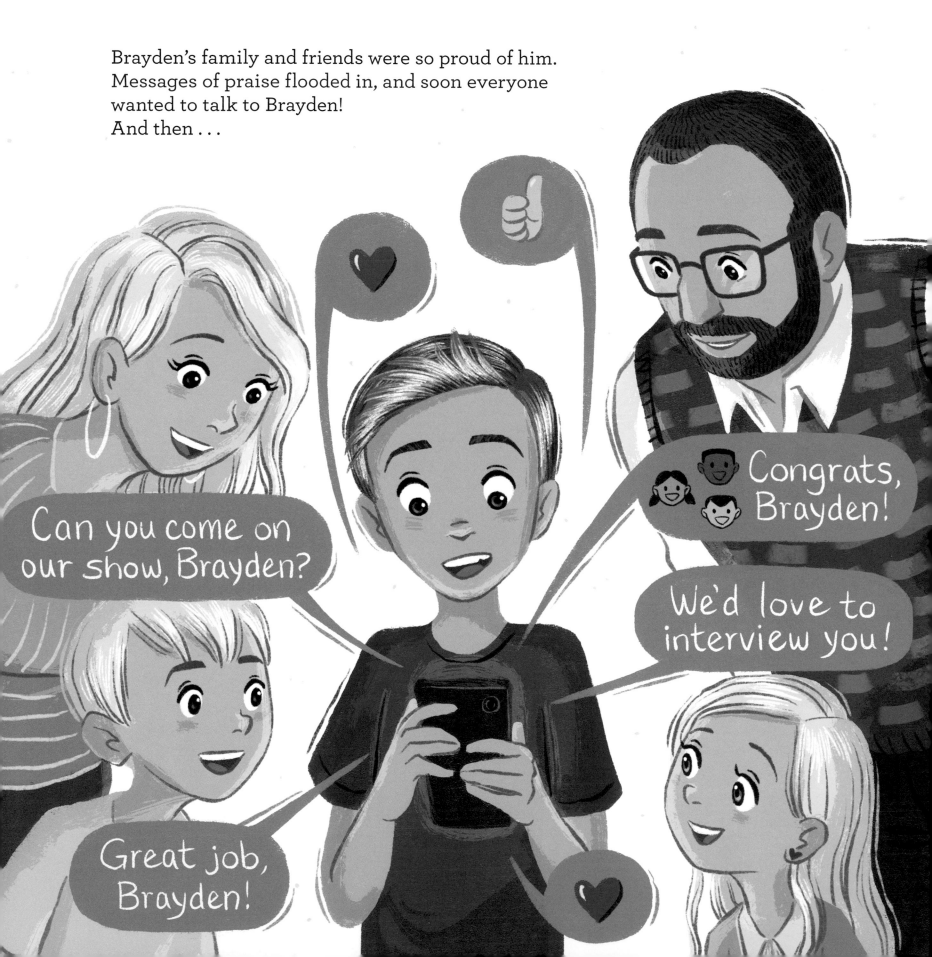

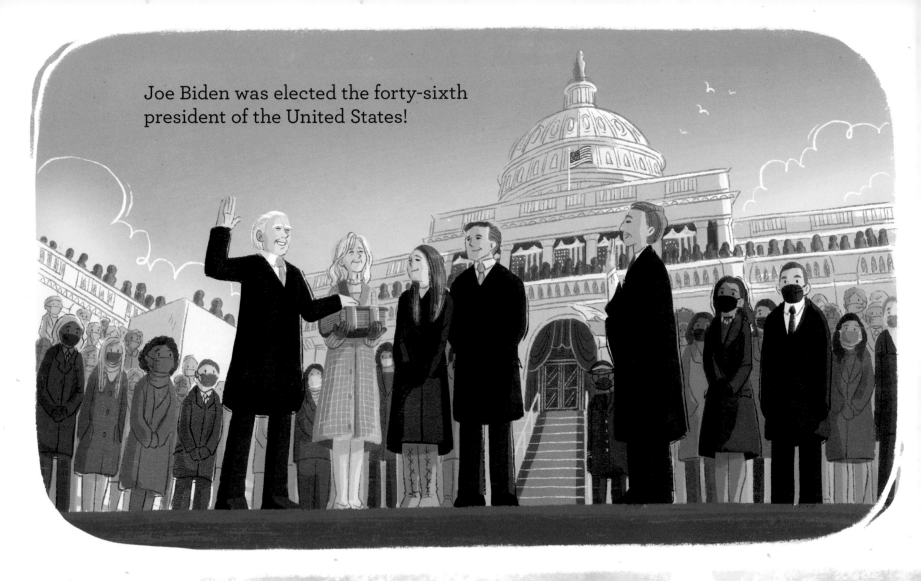

Joe Biden was elected the forty-sixth president of the United States!

President Biden asked his friend Brayden to join the celebration of his inauguration. This time, Brayden didn't hesitate. With great excitement, he recited President John F. Kennedy's immortal words: "Ask not what your country can do for you. Ask what you can do for your country."

The whole world applauded.

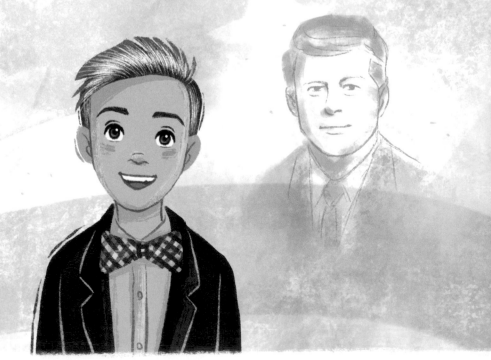

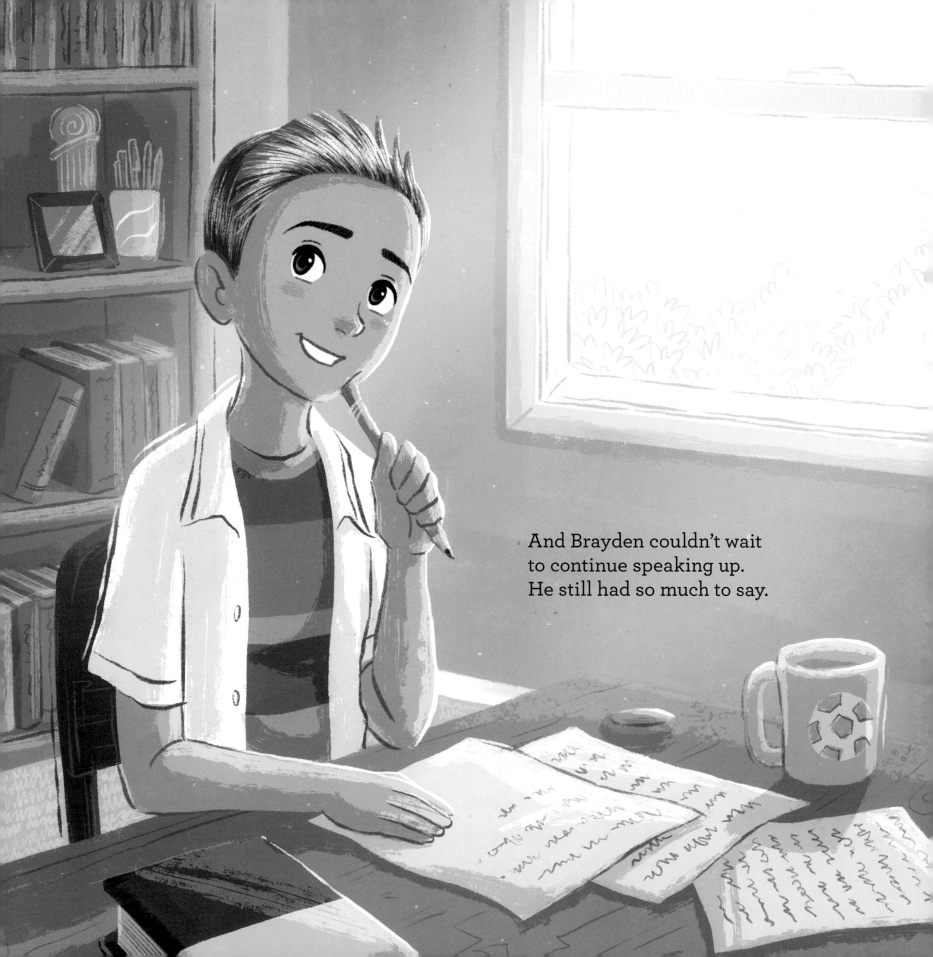

And Brayden couldn't wait
to continue speaking up.
He still had so much to say.

A NOTE FROM BRAYDEN

Sometimes, my bumpy speech made me uncomfortable.
I used to think everyone had to speak smoothly. Without bumps.

But there's nothing wrong with the way I speak. I have bumpy speech— and that's okay.

I hope other kids reading this won't feel embarrassed or ashamed if they stutter.

I know it's hard.

But you should feel good about the way you speak, even if it is bumpy.

And like the 46th president of the United States, Mr. Biden, you're a part of a pretty cool club— the Bumpy Speech Club.

So don't be scared to speak up, speak out, and use your voice. You are amazing just the way you are!

Brayden Harrington

Children who stutter:

- You are not alone.
- There are roughly 70 million people who stutter worldwide.
- No one speaks perfectly. Everyone has some level of "bumpy speech" throughout their lives.

Parents of children who stutter:

- You are not alone.
- As soon as possible, make sure your child is aware that they are not alone as a person who stutters. There are so many associations that will help. Some examples are the Stuttering Association of the Young (SAY), Friends: The National Association of Young People Who Stutter, the Stuttering Foundation of America, and the National Stuttering Association. All of these organizations will work with families to help children who stutter understand they are not alone and help them begin their journey of acceptance and understanding of stuttering. These organizations provide remote meetings as well as in-person conferences for children (and adults who stutter) to meet and share their experiences, challenges, and triumphs with stuttering.
- Your child does not need to fix their stuttering. Help them focus on acceptance and let them determine on their own whether they would like to use various strategies to minimize their stutter.
- Find a speech pathologist who will help with both strategies to work through a stutter as well as provide support toward acceptance of their stutter.
- Be as patient as possible. The sooner a child who stutters realizes they are perfect as they are, the quicker they will begin their journey of acceptance.
- Your local school system should be a source of support. This can start as early as three years old.
- Let your child pick the topic of conversation.
- Speak at a normal to slow rate.

Teachers of children who stutter:

- Be patient and accepting.
- Create a classroom community of acceptance so children who stutter are confident to share and speak out.
- Create a system of cues with the child who stutters to determine when they are comfortable enough to share. Allow the child to be your guide in this process.
- Use the above-mentioned organizations as a resource.

Above all, remember this quote:

"I look at stuttering as my gift."

Brayden Harrington realized this after he saw the impact he was able to make when he did not allow his stutter to define him. He spoke in front of the nation at both the 2020 Democratic National Convention and the Celebration of America portion of the inauguration of President Joe Biden.